BREAKING THROUGH CANCER

A Guide to Multiple Myeloma

Detailed Exploration of Causes,
Treatments, and Survival Strategies

Oliver Reminisce

Copyright © **Oliver Reminisce, *2024*.**

All rights reserved. No part of this publication may be reproduced, distributed, or transmitted in any form or by any means, including photocopying, recording, or other electronic or mechanical methods, without the prior written permission of the publisher, except in the case of brief quotations embodied in critical reviews and certain other noncommercial uses permitted by copyright law.

Table of Contents

Introduction 3
Chapter 1 5
   Understanding Multiple Myeloma 5
Chapter 2 8
   Causes and Risk Factors 8
Chapter 3 11
   Recognizing the Symptoms 11
Chapter 4 15
   Diagnostic Procedures 15
Chapter 5 20
   Prognosis and Survival Rates 20
Chapter 6 23
   Treatment Options 23
Chapter 7 28
   Managing Side Effects 28
Chapter 8 31
   Maintenance Therapy and Remission 31
Chapter 9 35
   Complications and Ongoing Care 35
Chapter 10 39
   Navigating the Healthcare System 39
Conclusion 44

Chapter 1
Understanding Multiple Myeloma

In the intricate world of human health, multiple myeloma stands out as a complex and formidable adversary. To understand this disease, we must first unravel the nature of the cells it corrupts and the profound effects it has on the body. At its core, multiple myeloma is a type of blood cancer that primarily affects plasma cells, a specialized group of white blood cells essential for our immune system's defense against pathogens.

Plasma cells are produced in the bone marrow, the spongy tissue inside our bones that acts as a production line for various blood cells. These cells are integral to the immune system, tasked with the crucial job of producing antibodies. Antibodies are Y-shaped proteins designed to recognize and neutralize foreign invaders like bacteria and viruses, ensuring our bodies remain safeguarded against infections. However, in multiple myeloma, this system is disrupted in a dramatic and destructive manner.

In this condition, the plasma cells begin to multiply uncontrollably, leading to an overproduction of abnormal antibodies known as monoclonal proteins or M proteins. These rogue proteins accumulate in the bone marrow, where they wreak havoc. Their buildup impairs the marrow's ability to produce healthy blood cells, leading to a cascade of health issues. The presence of these abnormal proteins also contributes to the damage of the bone marrow and bone structures, causing the bones to become weakened and brittle—a condition often likened to osteoporosis.

The effects of multiple myeloma extend beyond just the bones. The kidneys, tasked with filtering waste products from the blood, struggle to cope with the overload of M proteins. This can lead to kidney damage or even failure, compounding the challenges faced by individuals with this disease. As the condition progresses, the impact on the body becomes increasingly severe, manifesting in a range of symptoms that reflect the widespread damage caused by the abnormal plasma cells.

Understanding multiple myeloma requires not just knowledge of its medical definitions and background but also an appreciation of how this disease fundamentally alters the body's normal functions. By comprehending how plasma cells function and how their corruption leads to such widespread issues, we gain insight into the challenges faced by those living with multiple myeloma. This understanding is crucial, as it lays the foundation for exploring the treatment options and strategies that can help manage and mitigate the effects of this challenging disease.

As we move forward, we will continue to explore the complexities of multiple myeloma, delving into its causes, symptoms, and the latest advancements in treatment. Our goal is to provide a comprehensive view that not only informs but also empowers those affected by this disease, offering hope and actionable insights in the fight against multiple myeloma.

Chapter 2
Causes and Risk Factors

As we journey deeper into the realm of multiple myeloma, we encounter a crucial aspect of understanding this complex disease: its causes and risk factors. Despite the advances in medical science, the definitive cause of multiple myeloma remains elusive. The disease's multifaceted nature suggests that both genetic and environmental factors play a role, though no single factor can be pinpointed as the sole cause.

Multiple myeloma does not arise from a single, identifiable cause but rather from a combination of factors that disrupt the normal function of plasma cells. The search for a concrete cause is ongoing, but researchers have identified several potential contributors to the development of this disease.

Genetic predisposition is one area of significant interest. Although multiple myeloma is not generally considered a hereditary disease, certain genetic variations may increase susceptibility. Individuals with a family history of multiple myeloma or related blood cancers may face a higher risk, indicating that genetic factors can influence the likelihood of developing the disease. However, it is essential to note that having a family history does not guarantee that an individual will develop multiple myeloma, nor does the absence of such a history preclude the disease.

Environmental factors also play a crucial role in the risk profile for multiple myeloma. Exposure to certain chemicals and substances has been linked to an increased risk of developing this cancer. Notable among these is Agent Orange, a herbicide used extensively during the Vietnam War. Studies have shown a correlation between exposure to Agent Orange and a higher incidence of multiple myeloma. Additionally, excessive radiation exposure, such as that from repeated medical imaging or radiation therapy for other conditions, has been associated with an elevated risk of developing multiple myeloma.

The demographic factors further refine the understanding of multiple myeloma's risk profile. The disease is more commonly diagnosed in older adults, with the average age of diagnosis around 69. This age-related prevalence suggests that the cumulative effects of various risk factors over time may contribute to the development of the disease.

Additionally, demographic studies indicate a higher incidence of multiple myeloma in individuals of African descent. Research shows that African Americans are twice as likely to develop multiple myeloma compared to Caucasians. This disparity points to the potential role of genetic and environmental interactions unique to different populations.

While the exact interplay of these factors remains complex, the current understanding underscores the importance of both genetic and environmental components in the risk of developing multiple myeloma. Ongoing research continues to explore these factors in greater detail, with the hope of uncovering more precise causes and improving strategies for prevention and early detection.

By delving into these causes and risk factors, we gain a deeper appreciation of the multifaceted nature of multiple myeloma. This knowledge not only enhances our understanding of the disease but also informs ongoing efforts to mitigate risks and develop more effective treatments. As we continue to explore this topic, we move closer to unraveling the intricate web of influences that contribute to the onset of multiple myeloma, paving the way for better prevention and intervention strategies.

Chapter 3
Recognizing the Symptoms

In the labyrinth of multiple myeloma, recognizing the symptoms is akin to deciphering a complex code that reveals the presence of this elusive disease. Understanding these symptoms is crucial for early detection and effective management. Multiple myeloma, a condition characterized by the abnormal proliferation of plasma cells, manifests through a variety of symptoms that can often be mistaken for other health issues. This chapter sheds light on the key symptoms associated with multiple myeloma and introduces the CRAB criteria, a vital tool for diagnosing the disease.

The symptoms of multiple myeloma are diverse and can significantly impact a person's quality of life. Commonly reported symptoms include anemia, which can cause persistent fatigue, pallor, and shortness of breath. This is often coupled with bone pain, especially in the back and ribs. The pain is typically described as a dull, aching sensation that can worsen over time, leading to frequent fractures even from minimal trauma. Such fractures, particularly in the spine, may result in noticeable changes in posture or height.

Bleeding and bruising easily are also prevalent symptoms, stemming from the impaired production of platelets, which are crucial for blood clotting. This can lead to frequent nosebleeds, gum bleeding, or unexplained bruising. Alongside these, fatigue and weakness become prominent, as the body struggles to cope with the anemia and the general strain of the disease. Breathing difficulties and persistent nausea may also occur, further complicating the clinical picture.

In addition to these common symptoms, the CRAB criteria provide a structured way to understand the disease's impact on the body. The acronym CRAB stands for Calcium, Renal failure, Anemia, and Bone damage, each representing a significant aspect of the disease's progression.

Calcium Levels (Hypercalcemia): Multiple myeloma often leads to high levels of calcium in the blood, a condition known as hypercalcemia. This occurs when myeloma cells disrupt normal bone metabolism, causing calcium to be released into the bloodstream. Symptoms of hypercalcemia can range from subtle changes like loss of appetite and mild nausea to more severe manifestations such as confusion, excessive thirst, and kidney problems.

Renal Failure: The accumulation of M proteins, produced by the abnormal plasma cells, can overwhelm the kidneys' ability to filter waste. This leads to renal failure, which may present as increased thirst, frequent urination, or swelling in the legs and ankles. In severe cases, it may require dialysis to manage.

Anemia: Anemia in multiple myeloma results from the replacement of healthy bone marrow cells with myeloma cells. This reduces the production of red blood cells, leading to symptoms such as weakness, dizziness, and pallor. The reduced capacity to carry oxygen can cause shortness of breath and a general feeling of fatigue.

Bone Damage: The destructive impact of myeloma cells on bone tissue results in increased bone fragility and pain. This can manifest as severe back pain, bone fractures, or skeletal deformities. As the disease progresses, the risk of spinal compression fractures and other bone-related issues increases.

In addition to the CRAB criteria, it's important to consider the increased susceptibility to infections that patients with multiple myeloma face. The disease impairs the immune system, leaving individuals more vulnerable to bacterial, viral, and fungal infections. Persistent or recurrent infections, despite treatment, are a significant concern and require careful management.

Recognizing these symptoms and understanding their implications is crucial for the timely diagnosis and management of multiple myeloma. Early detection can significantly improve the effectiveness of treatment and enhance the quality of life for those affected. As we delve further into this disease, the goal is to equip readers with the knowledge to identify these symptoms and seek appropriate medical attention, paving the way for better outcomes and improved patient care.

Chapter 4
Diagnostic Procedures

In the journey toward diagnosing multiple myeloma, various procedures and tests play an essential role in confirming the presence of the disease and determining its progression. Early diagnosis can be challenging, as symptoms often overlap with other conditions, but modern diagnostic techniques allow doctors to paint a clearer picture of what's happening inside the body. This chapter delves into the key diagnostic methods and the significance of staging in understanding the severity of multiple myeloma.

Multiple myeloma can be identified through a variety of diagnostic tests, with blood and urine tests often serving as the first step. These tests can reveal the presence of abnormal proteins, such as M proteins, which are produced by myeloma cells. One common blood test used is the serum protein electrophoresis (SPEP), which helps to detect the abnormal antibodies. Additionally, the presence of free light chains can be found through specific assays, indicating the possibility of myeloma. Another key indicator is the level of beta-2 microglobulin in the blood, which can give insights into the disease's progression. Urine tests can also be helpful, particularly in identifying Bence-Jones proteins, another type of abnormal protein associated with multiple myeloma.

For a more definitive diagnosis, a bone marrow biopsy is usually required. During this procedure, a small sample of bone marrow is extracted, typically from the hip bone, and analyzed under a microscope. This allows doctors to assess the percentage of plasma cells present in the marrow. In patients with multiple myeloma, the bone marrow often contains a higher-than-normal concentration of these abnormal plasma cells. A bone marrow biopsy not only confirms the diagnosis but also helps in understanding the extent of the disease.

Imaging tests also play a crucial role in diagnosing multiple myeloma. X-rays are often used to check for bone damage, as myeloma cells can weaken bones and cause fractures. However, more advanced imaging techniques, such as magnetic resonance imaging (MRI), computed tomography (CT) scans, and positron emission tomography (PET) scans, provide a clearer and more detailed view of the bones and the extent of the disease. MRI scans are particularly useful for detecting myeloma lesions in the spine, while PET scans can help locate areas of increased metabolic activity, often associated with cancerous growths.

Once a diagnosis is made, understanding the stage of multiple myeloma is critical in determining the prognosis and planning the appropriate course of treatment. Multiple myeloma is typically classified into three stages based on the Revised International Staging System (R-ISS).

In **Stage 1**, patients usually have lower levels of the abnormal proteins, and the disease may not yet have caused significant damage to bones or other organs. The outlook for patients diagnosed at this stage tends to be more favorable, with treatments often being more effective in controlling the disease.

Stage 2 represents an intermediate phase, where the levels of proteins in the blood have increased, and some damage to bones or organs may be evident. At this stage, the disease is more aggressive, and treatment plans may need to be adjusted to manage the growing impact of the condition.

Stage 3 is the most advanced form of multiple myeloma, where high levels of abnormal proteins are present, and significant damage to the bones, kidneys, or other organs has occurred. Patients at this stage often experience severe symptoms and may require more intensive treatment to manage the disease.

In addition to the staging system, multiple myeloma can also be classified using **subtypes A and B**. Type A indicates normal kidney function, whereas Type B suggests some level of kidney impairment. This classification helps doctors better understand how the disease is affecting the kidneys and guides the approach to treatment, especially in managing complications like renal failure.

Before the full-blown development of multiple myeloma, there are premalignant conditions to be aware of. **Monoclonal Gammopathy of Undetermined Significance (MGUS)** is a condition in which abnormal M proteins are present in the blood, but the individual does not experience symptoms. While MGUS doesn't require treatment, it's a risk factor for developing multiple myeloma in the future. Monitoring is important, as about 1% of patients with MGUS progress to myeloma each year. **Smoldering myeloma** represents a more advanced stage than MGUS, with higher levels of abnormal plasma cells and M proteins, but without the organ damage or symptoms typically associated with active multiple myeloma. Like MGUS, smoldering myeloma requires regular monitoring to detect progression.

These diagnostic procedures and the classification of multiple myeloma stages form the backbone of the diagnosis and management process. Understanding them allows patients and their families to grasp the severity of the disease and the urgency of treatment, setting the stage for the decisions that follow. By knowing where they stand in terms of disease progression, patients can make more informed choices about their healthcare and treatment options.

Chapter 5
Prognosis and Survival Rates

In the realm of multiple myeloma, understanding prognosis and survival rates provides crucial insight into what patients and their families can expect in the journey ahead. Prognosis is not just about statistical survival rates but also involves understanding the factors that influence long-term outcomes, the impact of early detection, and the ongoing research aimed at improving treatment and survival rates.

Current Prognostic Outlook

Multiple myeloma is considered a chronic disease, with significant advancements in treatment extending life expectancy for many patients. Despite these advancements, it is generally not considered curable, and the focus remains on managing the disease effectively and improving quality of life. The overall survival rate for multiple myeloma patients has improved considerably over the past decades, thanks to better treatments and a deeper understanding of the disease. According to the American Society of Clinical Oncology, the five-year survival rate for multiple myeloma patients stands at approximately 58%. This statistic varies significantly based on the stage of the disease at diagnosis and the effectiveness of the treatment regimen.

For those diagnosed at an early stage, the outlook is more favorable, with a five-year survival rate of about 79%. Early detection is crucial in these cases, as it allows for the initiation of treatment before the disease has a chance to advance significantly. The impact of early detection cannot be overstated; it often translates into a better response to treatment, fewer complications, and an overall improvement in survival outcomes.

Understanding Long-term Outcomes

Long-term outcomes in multiple myeloma are influenced by various factors, including the stage at diagnosis, response to treatment, and individual patient characteristics. Even after achieving remission, patients must remain vigilant, as multiple myeloma has a tendency to relapse. The potential for relapse is a significant concern and underscores the importance of ongoing monitoring and follow-up care. Remission may be complete or partial, and while some patients may experience long periods of remission, others may face recurrence within a few years.

Relapse can occur for several reasons, including the development of drug resistance or the presence of residual disease that was not eradicated by initial treatments. Advances in treatment, such as new drug therapies and stem cell transplants, have improved the ability to manage relapses effectively, but they also present their own set of challenges and potential side effects.

The Role of Ongoing Research

Research continues to play a vital role in enhancing the prognosis for multiple myeloma patients. Scientists and clinicians are constantly exploring new treatment options, refining existing therapies, and striving to understand the underlying mechanisms of the disease better. Ongoing research efforts aim to improve survival rates, minimize side effects, and potentially discover a cure.

Clinical trials are a crucial component of this research, offering patients access to cutting-edge treatments and contributing to the development of new therapies. These trials help to assess the efficacy and safety of novel treatments, providing valuable data that can lead to more effective management strategies for multiple myeloma.

Additionally, research into personalized medicine, which tailors treatment to the individual characteristics of each patient, holds promise for improving outcomes. By understanding the genetic and molecular profile of a patient's disease, doctors can select treatments that are more likely to be effective and minimize the risk of adverse effects.

Chapter 6
Treatment Options

When it comes to managing multiple myeloma, the treatment landscape has evolved considerably, offering a range of options tailored to the individual needs of patients. The approach to treatment typically involves an initial phase of therapy to induce remission, followed by considerations for stem cell transplantation and, in some cases, CAR T-cell therapy. Each of these treatments comes with its own set of benefits, challenges, and procedural details, which are crucial for understanding how to effectively combat this complex disease.

Initial Treatment

The journey often begins with induction therapy, aimed at reducing the number of myeloma cells to a level where they are no longer detectable or cause significant symptoms. This phase of treatment is critical as it sets the foundation for subsequent therapy and helps determine the overall management strategy.

Induction therapy typically involves a combination of medications, each playing a specific role in attacking the myeloma cells and managing symptoms. Commonly used drugs include:

- **Lenalidomide**: This medication works by enhancing the immune system's ability to fight cancer and inhibiting the growth of myeloma cells. It is part of a class of drugs known as immunomodulatory agents, which are effective in managing multiple myeloma.
- **Dexamethasone**: A corticosteroid that reduces inflammation and suppresses the immune system, helping to control myeloma. It also alleviates some of the side effects associated with other treatments.
- **Carfilzomib**: This proteasome inhibitor blocks the breakdown of proteins within myeloma cells, leading to their death. It is a potent drug that targets the cell's protein degradation pathway, which is crucial for the survival of cancer cells.
- **Daratumumab**: Used in combination therapies, this drug targets the CD38 protein on myeloma cells, marking them for destruction by the immune system. Its inclusion in quadruple-drug regimens represents a significant advancement in treatment.

Stem Cell Transplantation

For many patients, the next step in treatment is a stem cell transplant, particularly if the disease responds well to initial therapy. The goal of this procedure is to restore the bone marrow's ability to produce healthy blood cells following high-dose chemotherapy that targets cancerous cells.

- **Process and Procedures**: The procedure begins with the collection of stem cells, typically from the patient's own blood or bone marrow. These cells are then frozen and stored while the patient undergoes high-dose chemotherapy, which aims to eradicate the myeloma cells. After chemotherapy, the stored stem cells are reinfused into the patient's bloodstream, where they migrate back to the bone marrow and begin to regenerate healthy blood cells. The entire process usually involves several weeks of treatment and recovery, often requiring a hospital stay.
- **Risks and Benefits of Autologous Transplants**: Autologous stem cell transplants, which use the patient's own stem cells, offer the benefit of avoiding complications associated with donor transplants, such as graft-versus-host disease. However, the procedure is not without risks. High-dose chemotherapy can lead to severe side effects, including increased susceptibility to infections, bleeding, and anemia. Additionally, the recovery period can be challenging, with potential long-term effects on organ function and overall health.

CAR T-cell Therapy

CAR T-cell therapy represents a cutting-edge approach to treating multiple myeloma, utilizing the body's own immune system in a novel way. This therapy involves modifying T-cells to better target and destroy cancer cells.

- **Explanation and Phases of Treatment**: The process begins with collecting T-cells from the patient's blood through a procedure known as leukapheresis. These cells are then engineered in a laboratory to express chimeric antigen receptors (CARs) that specifically target the BCMA protein found on the surface of myeloma cells. Once modified, the T-cells are multiplied in the lab and then infused back into the patient's bloodstream. Prior to infusion, patients typically undergo chemotherapy to prepare their immune system for the CAR T-cells, enhancing their effectiveness.
- **Potential Benefits and Challenges**: CAR T-cell therapy has shown remarkable results in some patients, leading to significant responses and durable remissions. However, the treatment comes with potential challenges, including the risk of cytokine release syndrome (CRS), a severe inflammatory response triggered by the activation of CAR T-cells. Managing this

condition and other side effects, such as neurotoxicity, requires careful monitoring and intervention.

Chapter 7
Managing Side Effects

Navigating the journey of multiple myeloma treatment often involves dealing with various side effects, which can significantly impact a patient's quality of life. Each treatment option comes with its own set of potential adverse effects, making it essential to have strategies in place to manage these challenges effectively. Understanding and addressing these side effects can help maintain the patient's well-being and adherence to the treatment regimen.

Common Side Effects of Treatments

Treatments for multiple myeloma, including chemotherapy, stem cell transplants, and targeted therapies, are designed to eliminate cancer cells but can also affect healthy cells, leading to a range of side effects. These side effects can vary depending on the specific treatment and the individual's overall health.

- **Nausea, Vomiting, and Diarrhea**: These gastrointestinal issues are frequent side effects of many cancer treatments. They can be caused by the direct effects of chemotherapy on the gastrointestinal tract or as a reaction to medications. Managing these symptoms often involves a combination of anti-nausea medications, dietary

adjustments, and adequate hydration to prevent dehydration and maintain nutritional intake.
- **Weight Changes and Mood Effects**: Treatments such as steroids, including dexamethasone, can lead to weight gain, increased appetite, and changes in mood. Steroids can also cause mood swings, anxiety, and even depression. Addressing these effects may involve counseling, support groups, and, if necessary, medication adjustments to balance the benefits of the treatment with its side effects.
- **Fatigue and Blood Count Issues**: Fatigue is a common complaint among patients undergoing treatment for multiple myeloma. It can result from the cancer itself, the treatment process, or a combination of both. Additionally, treatments can affect blood cell counts, leading to anemia, increased risk of infection, and bleeding issues. Regular monitoring of blood counts and supportive therapies, such as blood transfusions or growth factors, may be required to manage these issues.

Strategies for Managing Side Effects

Effectively managing side effects is crucial for maintaining a good quality of life throughout the treatment process. Several strategies can help mitigate the impact of these side effects:

- **Medication Adjustments**: Adjusting the dosage or switching medications can help manage side effects. For instance, anti-nausea drugs, appetite stimulants, and medications to counteract diarrhea can be prescribed based on the specific symptoms. It's important for patients to communicate openly with their healthcare team about any side effects they experience so that appropriate adjustments can be made.
- **Lifestyle Changes and Supportive Care**: Incorporating lifestyle changes can significantly improve how patients cope with side effects. Eating a balanced diet, engaging in moderate exercise, and practicing stress-reduction techniques can help manage symptoms like fatigue and weight changes. Supportive care, including physical therapy, psychological support, and complementary therapies such as acupuncture or massage, can also play a role in alleviating side effects and enhancing overall well-being.

Patients should work closely with their healthcare team to develop a personalized plan for managing side effects. This collaborative approach ensures that both the disease and its treatment are effectively managed, ultimately leading to a better quality of life throughout the treatment journey.

Chapter 8
Maintenance Therapy and Remission

The journey with multiple myeloma does not end with the completion of initial treatments; it transitions into a crucial phase of ongoing management and monitoring. This phase involves maintenance therapy and strategies for achieving and sustaining remission. Understanding these aspects is vital for long-term success and quality of life.

Overview of Maintenance Therapy

Maintenance therapy is a critical component in the management of multiple myeloma, aimed at prolonging the periods of remission and preventing relapse. After the initial treatment phase, which may include induction therapy and possibly a stem cell transplant, maintenance therapy helps to keep the disease under control with lower-intensity treatments.

- **Medications Used**: Several medications are commonly used in maintenance therapy to manage multiple myeloma effectively:
    - **Lenalidomide**: This drug is a cornerstone in maintenance therapy due to its ability to enhance the immune system's ability to fight cancer cells and inhibit the growth of myeloma

cells. It has been shown to improve survival rates and prolong remission in many patients.
- **Bortezomib**: Often used in combination with other agents, Bortezomib works by inhibiting the proteasome, a complex responsible for breaking down proteins within cells. This action can lead to the accumulation of proteins that promote cell death in myeloma cells.
- **Ixazomib**: A newer proteasome inhibitor, Ixazomib is administered orally and can be used in combination with other drugs for maintenance therapy. It offers a convenient administration route and is effective in keeping the disease under control.

Achieving and Sustaining Remission

Remission is the goal of multiple myeloma treatment, signifying a period when the disease is under control, and symptoms are reduced or absent. Understanding and achieving remission involves both defining what remission means and employing strategies to maintain it.

- **Defining Remission**: Remission in multiple myeloma refers to the reduction or absence of detectable disease. It can be categorized into different levels:
  - **Complete Remission (CR)**: All signs of the disease have disappeared, and no myeloma cells are detectable in blood or bone marrow.
  - **Partial Remission (PR)**: There is a significant reduction in disease indicators, but some myeloma cells remain detectable.
  - **Minimal Residual Disease (MRD)**: Even when clinical signs of the disease are undetectable, very small numbers of myeloma cells may still be present.
- **Strategies to Prolong Remission**: Achieving remission is only the first step; maintaining it requires ongoing effort and vigilance:
  - **Regular Monitoring**: Continuous monitoring through blood tests, bone marrow assessments, and imaging helps to detect any signs of disease recurrence early. Regular follow-ups with the healthcare team are essential for timely intervention.
  - **Adherence to Maintenance Therapy**: Consistently taking prescribed medications and

adhering to treatment schedules are crucial for sustaining remission. Any changes or disruptions in medication can affect the outcome.
- **Lifestyle Adjustments**: Maintaining a healthy lifestyle, including a balanced diet, regular exercise, and stress management, supports overall health and can positively impact disease management.
- **Supportive Care**: Engaging in supportive therapies and seeking counseling or support groups can help manage the emotional and physical aspects of living with multiple myeloma and contribute to maintaining remission.

Through dedicated maintenance therapy and a proactive approach to managing health, many patients with multiple myeloma can achieve long periods of remission and maintain a good quality of life. The ongoing collaboration between patients and their healthcare team is key to navigating this complex and evolving journey.

Chapter 9
Complications and Ongoing Care

Navigating the complexities of multiple myeloma extends beyond the initial treatment and remission phases. Patients must also be prepared to manage complications and engage in ongoing care to maintain their well-being and manage the disease effectively. This chapter explores common complications associated with multiple myeloma and outlines strategies for long-term care and monitoring.

Common Complications

Multiple myeloma can lead to various complications that impact a patient's quality of life and require careful management. These complications can arise from the disease itself or as side effects of treatment.

- **Bone Fractures and Kidney Failure**: One of the hallmark complications of multiple myeloma is bone damage. The disease often leads to weakened bones, making patients more susceptible to fractures. Bone pain and fractures can significantly affect daily activities and overall comfort.
    - **Bone Fractures**: Myeloma cells disrupt normal bone metabolism, causing bone loss and increasing the risk of fractures. Managing

bone health through medications like bisphosphonates or denosumab, which help strengthen bones, is a common approach. Additionally, ensuring adequate calcium and vitamin D intake can support bone health.
- **Kidney Failure**: Multiple myeloma can impair kidney function due to the accumulation of abnormal proteins and other factors. Kidney failure may necessitate treatments such as dialysis to help filter waste and manage fluid levels. Patients with kidney complications need regular monitoring and may require interventions to support kidney function.
- **Anemia and Its Management**: Anemia, a condition characterized by low levels of red blood cells, is another common complication of multiple myeloma. It can lead to fatigue, weakness, and reduced exercise tolerance. Managing anemia involves addressing its underlying causes and may include blood transfusions or medications like erythropoietin to stimulate red blood cell production.

Long-term Care and Monitoring

Effective long-term care and regular monitoring are essential for managing multiple myeloma and maintaining overall health. Ongoing care involves routine check-ups, monitoring for disease recurrence, and making necessary lifestyle adjustments.

- **Regular Check-ups and Monitoring**: Patients with multiple myeloma need to undergo regular check-ups to assess disease status, monitor for complications, and evaluate treatment effectiveness. Routine blood tests, bone marrow evaluations, and imaging studies help track the disease's progression and ensure that any issues are addressed promptly.
    - **Importance of Monitoring**: Early detection of disease recurrence or complications can lead to more effective interventions and improved outcomes. Regular visits to a healthcare team, including hematologists, oncologists, and other specialists, are crucial for maintaining health and managing any emerging issues.
- **Importance of Lifestyle Adjustments**: Adapting to life with multiple myeloma involves making lifestyle changes to support overall health and well-being. This may include:

- **Dietary Modifications**: A balanced diet rich in essential nutrients supports overall health and can help manage specific complications, such as bone loss. Patients may need to follow a kidney-friendly diet if kidney function is impaired.
- **Physical Activity**: Engaging in regular, moderate exercise can improve physical strength, bone health, and overall quality of life. Exercise programs should be tailored to individual capabilities and health status.
- **Stress Management**: Managing stress through relaxation techniques, counseling, or support groups can help improve emotional well-being and coping strategies.

By understanding and addressing common complications and committing to ongoing care, patients with multiple myeloma can better navigate the challenges of the disease and work towards a better quality of life. The collaboration between patients and their healthcare team is key to managing long-term health and achieving the best possible outcomes.

Chapter 10
Navigating the Healthcare System

Embarking on a journey through multiple myeloma treatment necessitates not only a comprehensive understanding of the disease but also adept navigation of the healthcare system. Effective management involves assembling a skilled healthcare team and utilizing resources to optimize care. This chapter delves into the essential components of building a robust healthcare team and highlights the advantages of dedicated myeloma centers.

Building Your Healthcare Team

The complexity of multiple myeloma demands a multidisciplinary approach to treatment, involving various specialists who each play a crucial role in managing different aspects of the disease. Constructing a healthcare team tailored to your needs is pivotal for receiving comprehensive and effective care.

- **Key Specialists Involved**:
  - **Hematologist/Oncologist**: This specialist is central to the management of multiple myeloma. Hematologists and oncologists diagnose the disease, prescribe treatments, and oversee the overall therapeutic strategy.

Their expertise in blood disorders and cancer is essential for guiding treatment plans and addressing complex cases.
- **Oncology Nurse**: Oncology nurses provide direct care to patients, administer treatments, and offer support throughout the treatment process. They also educate patients about their condition and manage side effects, ensuring that patients understand their treatment protocols and receive the necessary support.
- **Radiologist**: Radiologists perform and interpret imaging tests, such as X-rays, MRIs, CT scans, and PET scans. Their role is critical in assessing the extent of bone damage, monitoring disease progression, and detecting potential complications.
- **Orthopedic Surgeon**: For patients experiencing bone issues or fractures related to multiple myeloma, an orthopedic surgeon may be involved. They address bone-related complications and may perform surgeries to repair fractures or stabilize weakened bones.
- **Neurologist**: In cases where multiple myeloma affects the

nervous system, a neurologist may be consulted. They assess and manage neurological symptoms, such as pain or weakness, that can arise due to the disease or its treatments.
- **Nephrologist**: When kidney function is impaired, a nephrologist steps in to manage and treat kidney-related complications. They are crucial in cases of kidney failure, providing treatments such as dialysis and monitoring renal health.
- **Pain Management Specialist**: Managing pain effectively is a significant aspect of multiple myeloma care. Pain management specialists help alleviate pain through various methods, including medications, physical therapy, and other interventions.
- **Oncology Pharmacist**: Oncology pharmacists specialize in the medications used in cancer treatment. They ensure that drugs are administered correctly, manage potential drug interactions, and provide guidance on medication-related side effects.

The Role of Dedicated Myeloma Centers

Dedicated myeloma centers are specialized institutions that focus on the comprehensive treatment and research of multiple myeloma. These centers offer several advantages that can significantly impact patient care and outcomes.

- **Expertise and Specialization**: Myeloma centers bring together a team of experts with extensive experience in treating multiple myeloma. The concentration of knowledge and skills in these centers enhances the quality of care, as specialists are well-versed in the latest treatment protocols and advancements in the field.
- **Access to Latest Treatments**: These centers often have access to cutting-edge treatments and clinical trials that may not be available elsewhere. Participation in clinical trials can provide patients with opportunities to receive innovative therapies and contribute to research that may benefit future patients.
- **Comprehensive Care**: Dedicated myeloma centers offer a holistic approach to treatment, integrating various specialists to address all aspects of the disease. This comprehensive care model ensures that patients receive coordinated and efficient management,

addressing not only the cancer itself but also its complications and side effects.
- **Support Services**: Beyond medical treatment, these centers typically offer a range of support services, including psychological counseling, nutritional advice, and support groups. These services are crucial in helping patients cope with the emotional and practical challenges of living with multiple myeloma.

Navigating the healthcare system with multiple myeloma involves careful planning and collaboration with a diverse team of healthcare professionals. By assembling a skilled team and utilizing the resources offered by dedicated myeloma centers, patients can enhance their care and improve their quality of life. The synergy between specialized care and advanced treatment options plays a vital role in managing multiple myeloma effectively.

Conclusion

As we reach the conclusion of our exploration into multiple myeloma, it's essential to reflect on the journey we've undertaken. This book has delved into the complexities of this challenging disease, providing a comprehensive overview of its nature, causes, symptoms, diagnostic procedures, treatment options, and management strategies. Our aim has been to offer not just an informative guide but a source of hope and resilience for those affected by multiple myeloma.

Summary of Key Points

We began by understanding what multiple myeloma is—a cancer that affects plasma cells in the bone marrow, disrupting the production of normal blood cells and causing various health complications. From defining the disease to exploring its impact on the body, we covered the pivotal role of plasma cells, the production of abnormal M proteins, and the ensuing damage to bones and kidneys.

We then examined the causes and risk factors associated with multiple myeloma, recognizing that while the exact cause remains elusive, genetic and environmental factors play significant roles. This chapter highlighted the risk factors that could potentially increase susceptibility to the disease.

Identifying the symptoms of multiple myeloma is crucial for timely diagnosis. We discussed the common symptoms, including anemia, bone pain, and fatigue, and the CRAB criteria used to assess disease severity. Understanding these signs can lead to earlier detection and better management of the condition.

The diagnostic process involves a series of tests and procedures to confirm the presence of multiple myeloma and assess its stage. We covered the importance of blood and urine tests, bone marrow biopsies, and imaging techniques in diagnosing the disease and determining its extent.

Prognosis and survival rates offer insights into the outlook for patients based on the stage of the disease and the effectiveness of treatments. We explored how early detection can significantly impact long-term outcomes and the role of ongoing research in improving survival rates.

Treatment options for multiple myeloma include various therapies such as induction treatment, stem cell transplantation, and CAR T-cell therapy. We discussed each treatment approach, outlining the processes, benefits, and challenges associated with them.

Managing side effects is an integral part of the treatment journey. We provided strategies for dealing with common side effects and emphasized the importance of supportive care in enhancing the quality of life for patients.

Maintenance therapy and remission are key components of long-term management. We discussed the goals of maintenance therapy, the medications involved, and strategies for achieving and sustaining remission.

Finally, we addressed the complications associated with multiple myeloma and the ongoing care required to manage these issues effectively. From bone fractures to kidney failure, we outlined the necessary steps for long-term monitoring and lifestyle adjustments.

Encouragement for Patients and Families

Navigating the journey of multiple myeloma can be daunting, but it is also a path marked by hope and resilience. Understanding the complexities of the disease and the array of treatment options available provides a foundation upon which patients and families can build their strategies for managing the condition.

It is crucial to approach this journey with a spirit of perseverance and optimism. Advances in research and treatment continue to improve outcomes and offer new possibilities for those affected by multiple myeloma. The dedication

Printed in Great Britain
by Amazon